ADVICE FROM A
PARKINSON'S WIFE

20 LESSONS LEARNED THE HARD WAY

BARBARA SHEKLIN DAVIS

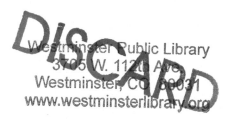

PARKER
HAYDEN
MEDIA

Dedicated to my husband, Leslie, who was my teacher.

INTRODUCTION

Living with an incurable disease like Parkinson's is very different from living with a terminal illness. This is a disease you're going to live with for a very long time. You really have to make peace with it.
— Connie Carpenter-Phinney, *Deseret News*, "Olympic cyclist shares his secrets to 'living well' with Parkinson's"

There are more than ten million people worldwide living with Parkinson's disease. Men are 1.5 times more likely to have Parkinson's than women. In married couples, a wife is thus statistically more likely than a husband to be a caregiver. Such is the case for me. I am seventy-five years old and my husband is seventy-seven. He has had Parkinson's for over twenty years.

I love my husband. In writing this book, I have no wish to hurt or embarrass him. He did not want to get

Parkinson's and he is not happy that he has it. There is no doubt that the burden of the person with Parkinson's is far greater than that of the caregiver. But the caregiver experience is not an easy one, particularly if the caregiver is a wife. Some have even suggested that the stronger the marital bond, the more difficult the challenge. My husband and I have been married for over fifty-five years. We have three wonderful children and nine delightful grandchildren. We both had fulfilling careers and enjoyed life. Parkinson's changed all that, not all at once, but gradually and inexorably.

Becoming a Parkinson's caregiver was uncharted territory for me. I am not particularly suited to the role by temperament, and certainly not by training. I remember telling a friend, whose husband had had the disease and recently passed away, that my husband also had it. She embraced me sorrowfully and said, "Oh, my dear. What a journey you are about to undertake." She was correct. Parkinson's is a journey with few signposts and few guides. Because the disease affects people so differently, because treatments that help one person are ineffective with another, because people are so different, it is very hard to generalize about Parkinson's.

But one thing I noticed is that Parkinson's spouses are not given much attention. Clearly the focus in the medical community must be on the patient; clearly the expectation in the larger community is that a wife will be there for her husband in sickness and in health, and vice versa. Thus, a Parkinson's spouse is somehow *expected* to know what to do, *expected* to bear the burdens without complaint, *expected* to be strong and capable and loving. But the Parkinson's journey is filled with the unexpected, and, in writing this book, I am hoping to provide others with some of the information and guideposts I wish had been available to me.

We live in an age in which transparency and authenticity are valued, and I think it is vitally important that people dealing with Parkinson's have as much knowledge and understanding as possible, in order to be intelligent about asking questions and making decisions, and realistic about meeting the challenges.

There are dozens of books that provide information about Parkinson's. In the age of social media and search engines, there are also many websites, podcasts, chat groups, and blogs about Parkinson's. But all of these, understandably, focus on the positive, on things that can be done successfully, on ways to manage, reasons to be optimistic, hopeful directions for the future. The result, however, is that many of the more serious and yes, depressing, issues tend to be glossed over. The really tough matters are discussed in scientific and medical journals, in a style and language that are inaccessible to the average person with Parkinson's or his or her care partner. Finding and reading these sources is a daunting task, and not really helpful to the layperson.

But caretakers need to know; they need to be prepared; they need to be informed. Most people are acquainted with the concept of caretaker burnout and caution caregivers to take steps to avoid it, but that does not take into consideration the fact that one's spouse is not going to die *from* Parkinson's, but *with* it, and the disease will be a part of one's marriage 'til death do you part. The Parkinson's spouse has to be knowledgeable. There was not a lot of information available to me when I began this journey two decades ago. Much more is available now, and the focus of these resources is on facts and understanding, as it should be.

This book, however, is different. It chronicles the serious matters that most Parkinson's spouses don't talk about publicly, the feelings and frustrations they are often ashamed to share. I hope that by speaking out, by revealing some of these issues to others, I can help them in ways that were not available to me, and let them know that they are not alone in dealing with the more negative impacts that Parkinson's will have on their lives.

It is well known that the spouses of patients with chronic or acute illnesses experience high levels of stress as a result of fear, uncertainty about the future, and the dramatic revisions they must make in their daily existence and in their long- and short-term life plans. But I found that one of the most agonizing aspects of being a Parkinson's wife was the feeling that I had no idea what I was doing and that no one could help me. For years, each time a new problem or symptom arose that seemed related to Parkinson's, I questioned the doctors and researched the internet, only to get no answers.

I struggled through alone, and it was only after having done so for a number of years that I began to find information online that validated my experiences and sometimes even provided helpful suggestions. Solutions don't always exist, but some comfort can be obtained through confirmation of your experiences and the knowledge that you are neither alone nor "making this up." This is particularly true with regard to the mental issues that Parkinson's causes, which are not as visible as the physical symptoms.

Family caregiving is still primarily gender-based. Women are the major providers of long-term care. Two-thirds of caregivers are female, and it is estimated that they spend as much as 50 percent more time providing care than their male counterparts. Men and women deal differently with caregiving responsibilities. Men tend to feel responsible for shouldering the financial burdens associated with long-term care and to work more or longer to meet these burdens. Women tend to stay home to provide hands-on care. As a result, women experience greater physical and mental strain and caregiver stress, exacerbated by social isolation and the reduction or loss of income from employment. This exacts a toll on their health, depresses their outlook on life, and increases their need for support. *Advice from a Parkinson's Wife* seeks to provide some of that support and to allow caregivers to understand that they are neither unaccompanied nor unappreciated in this role.

Parkinson's disease presents you with a whole new vocabulary. The average person has probably never heard, much less used, the words dystonia, bradykinesia, micrographia, and ataxia. But, as a Parkinson's spouse, these words become part of your everyday vocabulary. (They mean painful, prolonged muscle contractions; slowing down of movement; abnormally small, cramped handwriting; and lack of muscle coordination.) The actual manifestations of these words are part of your new life. Then there are other words, like hypomimia (reduction in facial expressiveness), camptocormia (bent spine syndrome) and sialorrhea (drooling) which you rarely encounter in the books, but which may very well define what you experience in your Parkinson's life.

Then there's the D word. Most people don't even associate dementia with Parkinson's, but it has been estimated that 50 to 80 percent of those with Parkinson's will develop dementia as their disease progresses. It takes about ten years from the onset of the disease for dementia to develop, but when it comes, it brings with it a burden that is far more difficult for the caretaker to bear than the physical challenges of Parkinson's. And you have to be prepared for all of this. That's what this book is for. Its goal is to share with you information and understanding of the experiences of the Parkinson's spouse and, in so doing, to make things easier and better for you.

I often think about my husband as he was years ago: he was a scientist, a chemist; he taught physics and computer science; he composed music; he played the bass; he was a photographer with a darkroom in our basement; he loved to go to concerts; he read Torah in our synagogue; he read science magazines voraciously;

he was an involved father; he loved expensive cars. Today he mostly sits and reads or he watches television. We still go to the movies and to the occasional concert. But he is not the man he used to be, and, as a result, I am not the woman I used to be. So many books and articles about Parkinson's promise hope, but there are no imminent advances in Parkinson's treatments. Maybe some day in the distant future there will be a breakthrough in this complex brain disorder, but for now, there is only acceptance and living in those moments when you can experience something approaching happiness, pleasure, and maybe even joy.

LESSON 1: ANOSOGNOSIA

It may well be our brains are wired up to be slightly more optimistic than they should be.
— Vilayanur S. Ramachandran, quoted in Errol Morris's "The Anosognosic's Dilemma"

CRASH! The whole house shook. I ran to the bedroom and found my husband on the floor. He had fallen off the bed as he dozed off watching TV. "I'm all right," he said groggily, as I got him back up. "Do you want to go to sleep?" I asked. "Yes," he answered so I tucked him in.

Getting up in the morning, I saw that the lights in his room were on, but I needed to go to the bathroom first. As I headed back to his room, I heard him calling, "Barbara, I need help." I found him flat on his back on the bathroom floor. "It's wet there," he said, although it wasn't. I got him to his knees and he pulled himself up using the handrails. I changed him and put him back to bed.

Two hours later, I was working at the computer and again, *crash!* I opened the bedroom door and found him face down on the carpet. "I'm okay," he said. I got him to his knees and got him up.

Later that day, our daughter came to visit and my husband commented, "I haven't fallen in a long time." "You fell last night and twice this morning," I said. "I did not!" he exclaimed angrily. He turned to our daughter and said, "I am concerned about involuntary falls, but I don't have any. I haven't fallen in a long time."

I used to think that Parkinson's patients were aware of their deficits and probably bothered and humiliated by the tremors, the drooling, the falling. And perhaps some are. But others are like my husband, completely lacking in self-awareness and any understanding of their disabilities and deficits, both physical and mental.

There's a name for this phenomenon: *anosognosia*. It means "lack of insight," and impairs a person's ability to understand and perceive his or her illness. It affects people with Parkinson's, Alzheimer's, schizophrenia, and bipolar disorder, which is why many who have these impairments do not seek treatment or refuse medication. Lacking awareness of their disease, they see no need for therapies. Studies of people with Parkinson's who have had deep brain stimulation and who are shown before- and after-surgery videos of themselves often express surprise at how disabled they were before the operation; they had no idea how impaired they were.

The blood is pouring down his leg from the cut on his knee where he fell. I'm trying to take off his pants and his shoes and socks. The dog is licking up the blood from the floor (yuck). My husband is giving me a hard time. "What are you doing?" he asks angrily. "I'm trying to bandage your knee from your fall," I answer. "I didn't fall," he says. I show him the bloody mess. "I didn't fall," he insists. I shake my head and continue the cleanup. "Get peroxide," he says.

Anosognosia can make life very difficult. If you don't acknowledge that you are likely to fall, that you do fall, that you fall often, you are not going to take steps to prevent falls. The anatomical damage caused by Parkinson's to the part of the brain involved in self-reflection makes denial of disability a way of life. That's why my husband still thinks he can drive, walk on the beach, swim in the ocean, and go on safari, while I am afraid to let him out of my sight or leave him alone for even a moment. That's why he avoids using the walker as often as he possibly can. That's why he falls so much. As frustrating as it is for me, it is equally so for him, since he sees nothing wrong with what he is and does, and can't understand why I am always so worried about him. Maybe it's a blessing; maybe it's nature's way of diminishing somewhat the awareness of how devastating Parkinson's is. But it definitely makes things harder.

LESSON LEARNED

The cognitive impairment of people with Parkinson's affects their self-perception; they simply do not realize how disabled they are. This complicates the caregiver's job, as she is perceived as offering assistance where none is needed.

HOW TO COPE

- Remember that this is a medical condition, caused by the deterioration of parts of the brain. It is not stubbornness or denial. Don't try to prove or insist on the person's limitations; this will only upset them and frustrate you. Instead, do your best to make changes discreetly, arranging things subtly that will help ensure their safety.
- Be compassionate and supportive. Even if the person with Parkinson's refuses physical therapy, "forgets" to use the walker, still thinks he can drive or travel to faraway places, he's not doing it on purpose. Be gentle and understanding, and try hard not to lose your patience.
- Allow them to do as much independently

as possible, while remaining alert and available to help. Find ways to help that preserve pride and above all, be patient. You understand what they are going through, even if they don't.

LESSON 2: THE BOOK THAT SAVED ME

What most doctors, even neurologists, don't realize is that while we use motor disfunction to diagnose PD, it is actually the behavioral problems that cause the most devastating consequences of this illness.
— Joseph H. Friedman, *Making the Connection Between Brain and Behavior: Coping with Parkinson's Disease*

DR. JOSEPH H. Friedman is Director of the Movement Disorders Program of Butler Hospital, and Professor and Chief of the Division of Movement Disorders at the Warren Alpert Medical School of Brown University, both located in Providence, Rhode Island. He serves as an Adjunct Professor in the School of Pharmacy of the University of Rhode Island.

Dr. Friedman is also the author of *Making the Connection Between Brain and Behavior: Coping with*

Parkinson's Disease, a book published in 2007 for people with Parkinson's, their families, and health professionals. This book saved my life and allowed my husband and our children to better understand the myriad symptoms that manifested in my husband's behavior and which were due to Parkinson's Disease (PD). I recommend this book unhesitatingly and with unqualified enthusiasm to every person I know who has a family member with Parkinson's.

Interestingly though, when I shared my excitement about the book with my husband's neurologist and suggested that he recommend it to his patients and their families, he was decidedly unenthusiastic. I guess that his interest was clinical and medical, and this book, even though written by a physician, was not sufficiently technical. Never mind that! This book will save lives— not the lives of PD patients, but the lives of their care-givers and families, who struggle on a daily basis without understanding what is happening to them. We can't all be physicians, but we can be informed patients and caregivers, and having a clear and informed under-standing of what Parkinson's is and does makes it infinitely more bearable.

Typically, the physician-patient relationship is characterized by what is known as "information asym-metry," that is, the doctor knows much more than the patient and takes the active role in the relationship, relegating the patient to a passive role. While the internet has rectified this imbalance in some ways, it is still the case that, in most medical situations, the physician knows much more than the patient. A great deal has been written about patient-centered care and making the patient part of the "care team," but the reality is (and should be) that the experts know more and that they communicate with each other in a language and syntax that are foreign to the average person. But patients and caregivers still need to know this information, and they need it to be accessible and pertinent to their daily struggles.

Today, there are a lot more books about Parkinson's; some are even better than Dr. Friedman's. And the internet is teeming with studies and advice and support. But I will always be grateful to this pioneering man who put knowledge and wisdom in our hands, when dealing up close and personal with this life-changing disease.

LESSON LEARNED

A great book can be a lifesaver. You can return to it again and again, and it will answer the questions you forgot to ask at the doctor's, the questions that arise as your Parkinson's journey progresses, and the questions you never thought could be asked, much less answered.

HOW TO COPE

- Buy *Making the Connection Between Brain and Behavior: Coping with Parkinson's*

Disease by Dr. Joseph H. Friedman. Buy extra copies for members of your family. (I have no connection with Dr. Friedman and make no money from this recommendation.) The book saved my life, and I hope it will do the same for you.

- Find other books and articles that are helpful. The Notes section of this book lists several, and your library will have others. Try to find a book that is of recent vintage and that is written in a style with which you are comfortable.

- The internet is a fantastic resource, from the latest research findings to ways of coping. You can Google any problem you have and you will find results. Some will not be helpful, but keep clicking. You're sure to find what you need. If you're searching in English, you may also find that the United Kingdom (Great Britain) and Australia are excellent sources, as they seem in many ways to be ahead of the U.S. in caring for people with Parkinson's.

LESSON 3: CLINGING

If the person with dementia clings to you and follows you around it can drive you to the limits of your patience. Not only does the person require your constant attention, but you are also deprived of even a moment's privacy. Moreover, it can be difficult to relax when you sense that the person is waiting for your next move.
— Alzheimer-Europe.org

I KNOW that I should react compassionately and kindly when my husband positions himself close—too close—to me on the couch and just sits there, doing nothing, saying nothing, but alert...watching, waiting. For what? Instead, I freak out. Inside. I try not to show it, but my personal space has been invaded, and every fiber of my being wants to get up and move to another chair. I know that would be mean, cruel, insensitive....so I sit there.....and fume inside.

I realize that my husband now lives in a world in which things don't always make sense to him, where strange people and animals appear, where anything could happen. He is dependent upon others and therefore at their mercy. This cannot be a pleasant experience, even though all his caregivers are compassionate, helpful, and kind. And even though I myself may not display those character traits at all times, I am nonetheless the one steady and reliable constant in his life. No wonder he doesn't want me out of his sight. Nonetheless, I can't live like this.

I feel guilty about creating busywork or setting him up with a television program, but it reduces his anxiety and my stress and makes me better able to cope with other things. Sometimes I hide magazines and pull them at times like this. "Look what just came in the mail!" I say. Other times, I ask him a question about things he is interested in (opera, chemistry, animals) and just let him talk. I can even move so I can face him instead of allowing him to crowd me. Of course, having to listen limits my ability to read or use my smartphone, but it works. He just wants attention. Sometimes I just try to disconnect from my surroundings, from his presence next to me, from my own need to attend to him and to be polite and inclusive. I notice that other people have little problem ignoring him, but it's much harder for me to do it. It's something I have to work on. It helps if I'm trying to read a really fascinating mystery.

It was helpful to me to learn that my reaction to this issue was not just due to my own personal failings as a care partner. A post on the website AgingCare.com let me know that I was not unique in my distress. It said that caregivers reasonably find shadowing and clinging "oppressive."[1] So while I may not be in the best of company, at least I know I am not alone.

LESSON LEARNED

The very real inability to function independently can lead the person with Parkinson's to a fear of being left alone. This in turn leads to clinging and following the caregiving spouse, which in turn provokes emotional distress and anxiety in him/her.

HOW TO COPE

- Recognize that you may be the only stable person in your spouse's constantly changing world. He truly needs you, even more than he knows, admits and appreciates.
- Deflect his attention by finding something for him to do. It doesn't have to be something that needs to be done or that needs to be done well. It just needs to occupy him for a while. It can be folding laundry, reading a newspaper, magazine or book, watching a television program or looking over old photo albums.

- Allow others to spend time with him. Invite one of his friends over for an hour. Hire a caregiver for several hours a week. Enroll him in a day care center. All of these will have the additional advantage of giving you a few hours of freedom for yourself, which will destress your life and make you better able to handle his constant need for contact.

LESSON 4: DOCTOR VISITS

In choosing a doctor, your major consideration should be how much the doctor knows and how well the doctor listens.
— MichaelJFox.org

YOU GO to see the doctor, or, just as likely, the nurse practitioner or physician's assistant once every six months for half an hour. That's one hour out of the 8,760 hours in a year. What do you do the other 8,759 hours? You're on your own. You're the expert. That MD, NP, or PA does not know your partner the way you do. The medical professionals don't see them when they're "sundowning," or confused or hallucinating or falling or stutter-stepping or accusing you of infidelity. In fact, your partner generally perks up for the visit to the doctor, appearing more alert, stronger, and more in command than he ever is at home. Not only does this make you feel ridiculous for raising issues and asking questions, but it gives the practitioner a false picture of what is going on.

My husband used to have a red Corvette, fulfilling the dream of a lifetime. We went to the factory to pick it up, and our name was up in lights over the factory door. He loved that car. But his driving was becoming erratic, as is the norm with Parkinson's. He constantly pulled off to the right, driving as much on the shoulder as on the road. As we veered off toward the guardrails, he would correct, but the whole process of veering and jerking back was alarming. One day he left for a dentist appointment and an hour later, the dentist's office called to ask where he was. Petrified, I stood deciding whom to call (police? hospital? 911?) when I heard the garage door open. He came in and told me he had gotten lost.... The EZ-pass bill that came later in the week showed that he had gotten on the thruway five times, driving in circles until he found his way home. But he insisted he could drive. "I haven't had any accidents," he said. That's how things stood when we went to the neurologist.

I was prepared to beg the doctor to tell him he couldn't drive anymore. Instead, he told the doctor about his red Corvette. "That's great!" responded the physician. "It's life-affirming!" I was ready to kill him. I don't know whose life was being affirmed, but I was definitely not ready for mine to be ended by my husband's driving.

It must be very difficult to be a physician for

Parkinson's patients. There's nothing you can do other than adjust their meds and measure their decline. You can't offer a cure or even much in the way of treatment except for deep brain stimulation; you can only watch them get worse. So it is no wonder that the doctor tried to be upbeat and positive and encouraging. You don't want your physician to give up on you and they don't want the patient giving up. But for the patient's partner, it's another story. How can you tell the truth about the patient's health and day-to-day living without sounding like Debbie Downer? How can you tell the doctor that your spouse can no longer dress himself, is incontinent, has trouble managing eating utensils, sees things that aren't there, and believes you are unfaithful when he tells the doctor that "everything is fine" and that he has no problems?

It's almost comical. The doctor asks, "Do you have hallucinations?" and he shakes his head no, and in the background I vigorously nod yes. "Are you still able to get around?" "Yes," he says. *No!* I silently yell as I shake my head. "Do you sleep well?" "Yes." *No*, unless by "well" you mean getting up several times a night, waking me up, and soaking the bedclothes. "How's your appetite?" "Fine." And I roll my eyes—he's lost thirty pounds, and I have to force him to eat every meal except dinner. But I don't say anything. I just hope the doctor sees me in the background steaming silently in contradiction.

LESSON LEARNED

You need to find a physician who listens to both the patient and the caregiving spouse.

HOW TO COPE

- A physician confessed online that when he enters an exam room, and a male patient has his wife with him in the room, "she is there to make sure I hear some part of his symptom history that he has never told me before."[1] He is completely correct, and it is vitally important that you make sure that the physician hears your voice.
- Speak up. Nonverbal messages are too easily ignored, especially if the physician is focusing on the patient, and the issues you are trying to raise are tangential to rather than directly related to the patient's condition, or are things the physician is uncomfortable talking about.
- Don't be afraid to change doctors. If your concerns are not allayed, your issues not addressed, or your questions ignored, it is time to find a new physician. And it is best to be honest about your reasons when you interview a new doctor; you don't want to go from the frying pan into the fire. You

have the right to have a doctor who is expert and experienced in the area of neuromotor disease but who also listens to and communicates well with both the patient and the caregiving spouse.

LESSON 5: FALLS

Around 70 percent of people with PD who fall do so recurrently and many fall very frequently.
— Natalie E. Allen, Allison K. Schwarzel, and Colleen G. Canning, "Recurrent Falls in Parkinson's Disease: A Systematic Review"

MY HUSBAND TOOK a six-week Falls Prevention course. Every time he went to the hospital, he received physical therapy as an inpatient, and for three weeks after we came home, he had outpatient PT. He was examined for strength, resilience, blood pressure, and balance each time we saw the neurologist. Here's what they found: he was very strong, his balance was above average, and his blood pressure from sitting to standing quickly resumed its proper level—sometimes it was hard to tell he had Parkinson's.

But he fell two, three, sometimes four times a day

with a terrified (and heart-stopping for me) yell each time. Each time the doctors asked him if he fell, he denied it. He refused additional physical therapy. I would sit there shaking my head in vigorous refutation of his statements. But they ignored me. I guess ignorance was bliss for them; they shared his state of denial. So I coped as best I could.

I adapted the environment to him: grab bars in the shower, rails on both sides of the stairs, walkers on every floor of the house, a wheelchair for when we went out. I moved furniture out of the way, bought a lift chair, adjusted the bed so it was easier to get in, got a kitchen chair with arms. But still, he fell.

I used to be able to go out for an hour a day, but he would inevitably take advantage of my absence to do something he used to and was no longer supposed to: make something to eat, load the dishwasher, search for a CD to listen to. And just as inevitably, I would come home to find him on the floor, sometimes cut and bleeding. It only took two of these episodes to make me stop leaving the house, even for the smallest errand, unless someone was there with him. But the falls continued, whether someone was there or not. I would be in the next room and hear him hit the ground. I could be five feet away and he would take a spill. For some reason, he rarely hurt himself—no broken hips, no broken ankles, no head injuries.

There are a number of studies of falls in patients with Parkinson's. Most people with Parkinson's who fall (which is most people with Parkinson's) do so a lot, up to seventy times per year. One interesting finding is that successful treatment of some symptoms may actually increase the number of falls because improved mobility increases the risk of falling. Another finding is that my husband's lack of serious injury is typical of Parkinson's patients, who generally fall indoors on soft carpet in what are known as "low-energy" falls because the patients walk slowly and fall from a low height. Whatever the case, the falls are stressful—perhaps more for the caregiver than for the faller. Maybe there's some special divine protection for Parkinson's patients, like for drunks in car accidents, although I doubt it. So I keep worrying and trying to keep him upright. It doesn't work particularly well.

LESSON LEARNED

Falls are endemic in Parkinson's. There is little you can do to prevent them, other than removing impediments to walking and installing bars and rails wherever possible. Constantly reminding the person with Parkinson's to move slowly, walk with heel first, carry nothing when they walk, and use the walker becomes tedious and has virtually no effect.

HOW TO COPE

- Fear not! Despite the dire statistics on the dangers of falling, the likelihood is that your Parkinson's partner will not injure himself, because he tends to fall slowly and not from a great height. Carpeted floors are advantageous; rugs are dangerous.

- When a fall occurs, keep calm and assess the situation. If the person is unhurt, allow him a few moments to recover his breath and his dignity. If he is hurt, call for assistance.

- The best way to help a person get up after a fall is to get him close to a solid piece of furniture which can support his weight. Have him get up on his knees. Do not attempt to lift him yourself. Bring over a chair if he is not near a bed or sofa; sit on the chair if you have to, to keep it from falling over. Allow him to slowly rise from his knees to a standing position and be ready with a walker or wheelchair once he is up.

LESSON 6: GUILT

The draining demands of caregiving and the uplifting effects of helping stand in apparent contrast to one another.

— Caregiving.org

A FRIEND whose husband has Parkinson's placed him in a nursing home. "I'm selfish, Barbara," she told me. "I want a life." I met another woman, divorced for over ten years, whose ex-husband got Parkinson's. She took him back to care for him. I understand them both.

I often think of the things I could be doing with my life: travelling to exotic places, going to interesting lectures, seeing shows on Broadway, having lunch or dinner with new and old friends, volunteering. The things I can do now are the things that can be scheduled between 10:00 A.M. and 3:00 P.M. two days a week, when I have an aide. And they have to be worked around dentist appointments, grocery shopping, car repairs, and other boring necessities of life. Then I think about how my husband wants to do things too: go to the opera, see the Grand Canyon, visit his children, swim in the ocean. He can't do these things any more than I can do what I want. So then I feel guilty.

People have suggested that I go to a support group. I resist for several reasons. The first is I have so much self-pity that I have little pity left to feel for others. The second is that when I have the time to get out of the house, I want to get away from Parkinson's disease, not spend an hour listening to others talk about it. Finally, I don't want to feel that I have it worse than others, or better, and commiseration won't make anything different. I don't mean to be cold, but I am selfish about my brief hours of respite, and I am only interested in finding practical solutions to my own situation, which no one else can realistically offer. But I still feel guilty.

It helps to know that there is something actually called "caretaker guilt." Caretakers are generally generous, kind, and loving people, but there is no question that, at some level, they want/expect/need recognition and appreciation of what they do. Often, with Parkinson's (or any chronic debilitating condition), this is not forthcoming. "Resentment is the caregiver's dirty little secret," wrote Lisa Hutchison, herself a Parkinson's wife. "When one is in a caretaking position long term, the expressions of gratitude may arrive less and less. A part of that is we get comfortable with one another.

Knowing that it is not intentional often does not erase the anger that is felt from being unrecognized."[1]

Then one day I found a very helpful quote online: "Unwarranted or inappropriate guilt truly serves no one. It will also suck the life and energy out of you. Refusing to be ruled by caretaker guilt is part of taking care of you!"[2] That woke me up. The site went on to say, "The caregiving journey is destined to be one of angst and suffering if you let guilt move in and stay. While you do not necessarily have to kick it all the way to the curb, caregiver guilt should at the very least be shown to the door." This made me realize that a Parkinson's spouse really does have more control over the situation than I had formerly believed. Hmmm. Maybe a support group is a good idea. Or I could call a hotline. Or write a book.

LESSON LEARNED

Guilt and caregiving go hand in hand.

HOW TO COPE

- Admit it. Own up to the resentment. You're entitled to feel it, because you are doing very difficult and challenging work. When you give yourself permission to feel guilty, and you recognize that your feelings don't have to control your actions, you will feel less guilt.

- Be selfish. You will be a more effective caregiver if you care for yourself. The Parkinson's patient may expect selfless service, but that is neither a healthy nor a realistic expectation. Caring for yourself will allow you to be a better caregiver and to provide better care for a longer period. You should not feel guilty about caring for yourself; it simply improves the care you provide for your spouse.
- Get help. Help with the house. Help with the spouse. Help in the form of a support group or a friend in a similar situation with whom you can commiserate. You are entitled to all of these things and should not feel an ounce of guilt about taking advantage of them.

LESSON 7: HOW YOUR MARRIAGE CHANGES

Martyrdom is overrated as a coping mechanism.
— Sotirios A. Parashos, Rose Wichmann, and Todd Melby, *Navigating Life with Parkinson's Disease*

THE AARP BULLETIN reported on a survey it took of five hundred doctors who regularly treat patients over fifty with dementia. The study revealed that 88 percent of the doctors said that when a patient has dementia, they feel as though they are treating two people—the caregiver and the patient. How right they are! No matter how much the Parkinson's patient suffers from the physical and mental afflictions caused by the disease, there is no doubt that the patient's partner is suffering too. Usually silently, usually guiltily, usually unnoticed by the patient.

The world of the Parkinson's couple is constantly shrinking, becoming smaller and more limited all the time. It's hard to get out. It's hard to find people who want to come visit you. It's hard to accept that you cannot do what other people your age do or what you expected to be able to do at your age. Or what you dreamed all your life of doing. Conversation between the Parkinson's couple becomes virtually nonexistent. The relationship changes from partnership to parenthood, only the baby is now really an adult and not nearly as cute as the genuine article. Drool, diapers, and feeding are much more fun when an infant or toddler is involved—not only are they sweet and cuddly, but they smile and giggle and give you reinforcement as you cope with the mess.

I never expected this life. I read recently that you can recognize a good marriage when each partner considers the other to be his/her best friend. I used to tell my husband everything; we had a good relationship; we agreed about most things. And I had a busy, active, and fulfilling life. I worked at jobs I loved, sometimes two or three at a time. I thrived on being busy and in charge and doing what I saw as meaningful work. Caretaking is very different. Certainly it is meaningful and important, and I am busy and in charge. But, to be frank, I hate it. I do not have the personality for it. I am frustrated, resentful, angry and stressed; I am ridden with guilt. He neither recognizes nor accepts how disabled he is. I can no longer talk with him, no longer tell him my troubles, no longer be understood or consoled by him. I have lost my partner.

There is no solution for these problems. Parkinson's

only gets worse, not better. So the only advice I ever give to others is don't put off for the future the things you want to do now. We had lovely travel plans, so many places we wanted to visit, experiences we wanted to share, people we wanted to see. Not gonna happen. There are still things we do: We go out to dinner; it's not elegant, but he likes it. We go to see shows; it's challenging when there is no wheelchair accessibility, but we do it. The movies are always fun, even though we leave huge popcorn messes all around us. And then there are holiday celebrations with family. That's the very best thing. I love to see him laugh with the kids and make wisecracks. The grandkids don't notice his deficits. In fact, they are even more pleased when he does something funny or smart *because* of his deficits. They are unfailingly kind and helpful.

I think you have to give yourself permission to grieve your marriage. The person you are wed to now is not the person you married. Your marriage now and in the future is not the marriage you had in the past. Hopefully, you have happy memories to look back on. But for now, it's best to accept that things will never be the same, and go through the trajectory of grief: denial, anger, bargaining, depression, and, ultimately, acceptance. We all hope at first that the diagnosis is wrong, then we get angry that it's happening to us. We bargain with the doctors or with a higher power, and we hope and pray for a solution. Then we get depressed as we realize that there is no solution. What's left is acceptance. Frankly, when you get to that point, things become easier. Your expectations diminish; your standards change. You realize that so much of what used to seem important (punctuality, entertaining, being well-dressed) is really insignificant compared to just having a full night's sleep, a meaningful conversation, a good laugh.

So do everything you while you still can, with people you love, even if you have to take loans out to do so. Live in the moment and make good memories now. You can pay back the loans over the years in which you will be unable to check things off your bucket list. At least you'll have nice photos on your phone for reminiscing.

LESSON LEARNED

As Parkinson's progresses, your marriage will change, whether you like it or not.

HOW TO COPE

- Whether yours was an egalitarian marriage or your spouse wore the pants, you will be wearing them eventually, and you'd better make sure they fit. If they handled the finances, for example, it is time for you to be 100 percent sure that you know what your income is, whether you have investments, what insurance coverage you have, and how to handle the taxes. If your spouse will share his knowledge with you, that is ideal. If, due to denial or the fear of losing control, they refuse to teach you what you need to know, find another way to learn it. Eventually, you will be in charge of the purse strings, and you must be informed and intelligent about doing so.

- It's okay to be sad about the losses. When you said, "I do," you never expected it to mean "I do everything," but now it does. So it's okay to mourn the loss of a partnership and to feel sorrow about what is lost and what has replaced it, but ultimately you just have to go on.

- Living in the moment and reliving fond memories can be joyful also. While you may not be able to do what you used to or what you had hoped to, you can recall the things you did. All those photos which you did (or did not) put in albums, all the slides, all the pictures on your cell phone can be shared with your spouse. Reminiscing is shared joy, and will remind you that your marriage is still meaningful and wonderful.

LESSON 8: THE KINDNESS OF STRANGERS

People are defined by core values and not by diseases.
— Michael Okun, M.D., *Parkinson's Treatment: 10 Secrets to a Happier Life*

SOME PEOPLE ARE AWFUL. Did the flight attendant really need to come over and tell us that in the event of emergency, we would be the last off the plane? What goes through the minds of hostesses at restaurants who say, "Have a nice evening," but don't move a muscle to open the door so I can push the wheelchair out?

But then there are the other folks, the kind ones. We live in the North, but the kindest people seem to live in the South. When we spend two winter months in Jacksonville Beach, Florida, many people offer to help me put the wheelchair in the car (no one has ever done so in New York). Southerners hold doors open or tell their children to run and open them. Some offer to carry things for me; some help my husband get up from a movie theater seat. It's truly heartwarming. They do it graciously and unselfconsciously. The North has more handicapped parking spaces and curb cutouts, but it has fewer people who go out of their way to be kind. "We're all in this together," said one Southern gentleman after helping us. What a wonderful way of thinking!

Parkinson's partners are often advised to ask for help. This is much easier said than done, and there's no guarantee that the requested assistance will be forthcoming. It's not that I blame other people. Taking care of a person with Parkinson's—even for an hour—can be a big responsibility. There is always the danger of falls. There is the lack of conversation, of responsiveness, of appreciation. There is the possibility that the person will become anxious and afraid, or freeze, or try to do something they shouldn't. Not only are the mental and emotional issues difficult, but handling a person with motor issues is also fraught with problems. It takes some level of experience and physicality to help a person with Parkinson's stand, sit, walk, eat, get into or out of a car, and into or out of a wheelchair. Not everyone is equipped to do this. Not everyone wants to help with these things. So while the books tell you to ask, they don't tell you how to deal with unwillingness, or willingness that falters in the face of reality. I'm afraid to leave my husband with just anyone, even if they are kind and well-meaning. Sometimes it only makes things worse.

All of which does not mean that I don't appreciate it when someone offers a hand, when friends ask us to have dinner with them at a restaurant, when people talk to my husband as a peer or a colleague, when they don't condescend, when they give him a little extra attention or tolerance because they see his condition. I'll never forget the restaurant manager who, seeing my husband struggle to scoop up food with his fork, wordlessly brought over a soup spoon. Or the kind baggage attendant who not only got us a wheelchair but changed our seats on the plane so my husband could sit farther up front. Or the waitress who brought him whatever he asked for, even if it wasn't on the menu, and called him "honey" and made him feel important.

I am grateful for the kindness of friends and strangers. Their core values define them.

LESSON LEARNED

It's hard to predict how people will react a person with Parkinson's, but in the majority of cases, people are kind.

HOW TO COPE

- Don't be afraid to disclose the disease.
  Some people instantly recognize that a
  person has a neurodegenerative disorder,
  either because they have had experience
  with it in a friend or family member, or
  because they are just sensitive people.
  Likewise, there are insensitive people who
  just don't seem to recognize that your
  spouse has a disability. Inform them. You
  can do it quietly, politely but firmly. Simply
  saying, "My husband has Parkinson's,"
  generally does the trick.

- Getting help is a mixed bag. While there
  are some people who are ready and willing
  to step up, there are others who are not.
  Some family members are eager to help,
  and others are reluctant. A willing helper is
  much better than an unwilling helper.
  That's what makes paid help easier in
  many ways. You have to try different
  options before you find the one that's right
  for you, and it may take a while before you
  get it right.

- When people are kind, thank them
  sincerely. People who help don't do it for
  the gratitude, but there is every reason for
  you to let them know how very special they
  are. And sometimes people just don't know
  how to help, although they would be

willing to do so. It's okay to ask them to open or hold a door for you or to move their chair to allow the wheelchair to pass. While you may get some disgruntlement, it's on them, not you.

LESSON 9: LET ME DO IT

I found that this Parkinson's does slow you down,
whether you want to slow down or not.
— Reverend Billy Graham

A FRIEND and her husband went to a niece's wedding
with her sister and brother-in-law, who has Parkinson's.
It was time to leave for the ceremony, but the man had
not yet buttoned his shirt cuff. Fifteen minutes passed.
It was past time to leave. My friend offered to help.
The man refused the offer. "Let me do it," he
responded. A half hour later, he was still struggling. By
the time they all arrived at the church, the young
couple were husband and wife.

Parkinson's patients' advocates tell them: don't let
people rush you. Take your time. Parkinson's advice
books and columns say: don't try to hurry them along; it
will only make things worse. But what happens when

you go to a restaurant and the server comes to your table for the third time and your spouse still has not selected an entrée? What do you do when you need to leave for an appointment and your partner has been in the bathroom for twenty-five minutes with no sign of imminent departure? When it takes ten minutes to buckle the car seatbelt?

They say that time is different for Parkinson's patients. Dopamine is the main neurotransmitter involved in time processing. The neurons that die in patients with Parkinson's disease are the very ones that control how the passage of time is perceived. Parkinson's patients, lacking dopamine, are unable to properly judge time. They significantly underestimate temporal duration, which means that they think time is passing much more quickly than it actually is. Five minutes to us seems like a minute to them. Thus, while they may take far longer to do things than people without Parkinson's do, they do not perceive this to be the case. And you have to adjust accordingly.

Psychomotor slowing is characteristic of Parkinson's. It involves a slowing down of thought and a reduction of voluntary movement. My husband always used to be in a hurry. He would start the car before I had even closed the door and buckled my seatbelt. He hit the gas pedal the minute the traffic light turned green. We were never late for anything. Parkinson's changed all that. Everything now takes two, three, or four times as long as it used to. Putting on shoes is a half-hour project. Eating breakfast takes forever.

Making a decision consumes hours. Yet at the same time, he still wants to hurry. He tries to get up fast; he tries to walk fast; if the doorbell rings, he leaps up to answer it. Impulsivity is another characteristic of Parkinson's, and it is a dangerous one because it can lead to falls.

Also among the many contradictory aspects of Parkinson's is that despite the overall slowness of their movement, Parkinson's patients also exhibit "motor hastening," typically when they walk. They start out slowly but speed up as they go, moving faster and faster in a gait known as "festination." Which is why, paradoxically, if I'm not telling my husband to hurry up, I'm telling him to slow down.

LESSON LEARNED

Everything slows down with Parkinson's. This is a challenge for those who do not have the disease.

HOW TO COPE

- Allow extra time for everything. It may start with fifteen minutes and become half an hour or more. Rushing is a thing of the past. "Hurry up" is a meaningless exhortation. Your spouse moves more slowly; he doesn't perceive the slowness. And the further the disease progresses, the less likely he is to be able to do things for himself as he used to, and you will have to do them. That slows it up even further. Anticipate the extra time and save yourself from the stress of hurrying.

- Make adaptations that will allow things to proceed more smoothly. Slip-on shoes take far less time than shoes that tie. A polo shirt takes less time to pull on than a shirt that buttons up the front. Print out the menu from the restaurant two hours before you leave the house and let him select what he wants. (Of course, the specials will mess this up!) Learn to do other things while he slowly accomplishes whatever task he is engaged with.

- Stop expecting quick decisions or action. Keep the choices as simple as possible. Ask yes or no questions. Thinking slows down as well as physical movement and you have to accept this and adjust accordingly. We all know that the world we live in tends to be too harried; maybe the blessing here is that Parkinson's slows it down.

LESSON 10: LITTLE PRACTICAL THINGS

It's not the load that breaks you down, it's the way you carry it.

— Lena Horne

THERE SHOULD BE a *Consumer Reports* for Parkinson's so you could find out which diapers, wheelchairs, feeding utensils, clothing, etc. are the best, most cost-effective, most efficacious. Trial and error is expensive and wasteful. Of course, I realize that every person with Parkinson's is different and what works for one might not work for another. That is true of any product, as one can see by reading product reviews, but here are some of the things I have learned the hard way.

1. An aluminum transport wheelchair is much lighter than a steel one. If you are putting it into and taking it out of the trunk of your car several times a day, the difference in weight makes a *big* difference. Also, if

you are buying a new car, try putting the wheelchair into it. I was astonished that it was much easier to put the wheelchair into the trunk of the Toyota Corolla I rented in Florida than into my big Honda CRV at home. Little things like that matter.

2. A transport wheelchair does not provide the most comfortable seating, but putting a small pillow on the seat can make a big difference. It's wise to pick a pillow in a washable fabric, as there will be food spills.

3. Unisex overnight diapers save you from having to change bedding and wash bedclothes, a difficult, energy-inefficient, and time-consuming task. It took me a while to find them, and I was reluctant to order them online, but the Amazon store brand made a big improvement in my life. I now use them during the day also. They hold a lot and don't leak. Depend® brand worked great for a long time, but their design emphasizes looking like underwear. Looks no longer matter to me—absorbency does.

4. There are a lot of cutlery options for people with Parkinson's, but they are mostly designed to minimize tremors. My husband does not have a problem with tremors; his difficulty is that his eye-hand coordination is poor, and he seems to have forgotten how to use a knife and fork. I don't know if there is anything out there to help with this, but I have learned that most restaurants (not all) will cut up his steak if you ask them to do so. I used to ask them to slice the meat, but now I even ask them to cut it into bite-size pieces. Ninety-five percent of the time they are amenable to the request.

5. Since my husband can no longer button shirt buttons, it became my job. A lot of things have become my job, and this was one that I did not relish. My daughter bought him a shirt with magnetic buttons that look just like regular ones. The shirt comes together in a jiffy with a series of cute little snaps and looks just like a regular shirt. It saves time and aggravation. (It also does interesting things in the washer, when the magnets stick to the tub wall, but if you snap it together before washing, it works fine.) Interestingly, my husband cannot take the shirt off by himself, although all it takes is one pull. Parkinson's is a very strange disease.

There are blogs and websites where people share "hacks" on adapting to Parkinson's and there's a book that lists three hundred things you can do to make life with Parkinson's easier. Most make a lot of sense, like putting handrails on both sides of a stairwell or putting food on plates of a contrasting color to make them easier to see. But you have to be cautious in implementing some of the suggestions; for example, satin sheets and tricot pajamas. One or the other works very well. But used together, they are a recipe for a *really* fast slide onto the floor.

LESSON LEARNED

There are lots of little tricks that make life with Parkinson's easier, but you have to look and listen hard to find them.

HOW TO COPE

- One of the best sources of suggestions are people who are in the same boat; that's why I wrote this book. But I am astonished at the instantaneous connection I always feel when speaking with another Parkinson's partner. We share experiences that are unique to each of us but also unique to the disease, and which nobody else can understand if they haven't been there. Also, there is no need to pussyfoot around problems or use circumlocutions when discussing matters that can cause others discomfort. If you have a professional aide, such as a healthcare worker or nurse, watch how they do things. Their training enables them to move a Parkinson's patient with greater efficiency, for example, and without hurting themselves. Most are happy to share their expertise with you, if you ask, and it will be very beneficial.

- If you can find a good gerontologist in your community, try to schedule an appointment. I found one late in the game, and it was so wonderful to talk to a doctor who completely understood what I was talking about with regard to my husband, who could explain what was usual and normal and who could, while not offering cures or answers, at least help me to better understand—and thus cope with—the myriad manifestations of Parkinson's disease.

- Always try to anticipate what you will need, and be prepared. You may not need to implement right away, but you will be ready when the time comes. The first time my husband started sloping off his chair, I bought Velcro straps to keep him upright. We didn't need them for many weeks, but when we really needed them, they were in the closet. Interestingly, we had to use them for a while, and then this symptom disappeared. Same was true for a bib, a dish with sloped sides, and bedrails. But at least I had these things on hand and didn't have to scramble when the need arose for their use.

LESSON 11: IS THERE SOMEBODY IN THERE?

In Parkinson's disease, masking can develop as the progressive loss of motor control extends to the facial muscles as it does to other parts of the body. Masked faces can complicate an already difficult situation, alienating acquaintances who may be put off or disturbed by the apparent lack of emotional response.
— Patrick McNamara, "Facial Masking in Parkinson's Disease"

I TOOK my husband to see a one-man comedy show. We were given seats in the front row of the small theater, because they were the only ones accessible to someone in a wheelchair. The comedian was pretty funny, but also a little high-strung and very aware of his audience, particularly those in the front row. At one point, he knelt down to my husband and asked, "Are you okay? You're not laughing." He quickly made another joke, and the moment passed. Had he been any more obnoxious, I would have said, "My husband has Parkinson's." That would have definitely killed his act.

Most people think Parkinson's means tremors. They have no idea of the whole conglomeration of symptoms, both physical and mental, that result from PD. And, of course, Parkinson's affects each person differently. But for many if not most, Parkinson's significantly impacts facial expression, speech, and body language. Facial masking means that you can't rely on what a Parkinson's patient looks like to know whether they are interested, happy, bored, depressed, paying attention, or out to lunch. Speech becomes quieter and harder to understand. PD patients may look like they're sleeping (open-mouthed, drooling, eyes closed) or they may just sit staring into space, seemingly oblivious to everything going on around them, when in reality their minds are fully functional, but their body language is all wrong.

This makes things harder all around. Do you ignore your spouse because they seem to be ignoring you? Do they then feel ignored and slighted because in their own minds they are alert and eager for your attention? Researchers have found that the facial masking caused by Parkinson's lends observers—including physicians—to see patients as more depressed, less sociable, and less cognitively competent that they really are. Flat affect, coupled with those negative impressions, leads people to avoid a person with Parkinson's. Toss in some apathy—another common

Parkinson's trait—and you have the recipe for unhappiness.

But who is cooking this recipe? Is my husband unaware that the reason I keep asking, "Are you all right?" and "Is something the matter?" is that he looks so miserable? Sherri Woodbridge, who has Parkinson's, says "Believe me, a person with Parkinson's is aware of their lack of expression."[1] So what is the Parkinson's spouse to do? Matt Townsend, a speaking coach and blogger, offers some insightful and practical suggestions for communicating with people who demonstrate flat affect. First of all, he notes that "when we're not getting feedback from others, we tend to take it personally," so the very first step is "Don't personalize their difference to be a reflection of you. Their lack of affect is no more your fault than your mother's love of strawberry ice cream is because of you."[2] He reminds us that "everything isn't always about you" and that "people are different, so just accept them as they are." I've also found that the best thing is to surround both of you with friends and family and to go to movies or concerts. You'll probably both enjoy yourselves, even if one of you doesn't show it.

LESSON LEARNED

One of the least well-known Parkinson's symptoms is facial masking, leading people to significantly misread the emotional states of people with Parkinson's, mistaking their frozen faces as depression, disinterest, or distress.

HOW TO COPE

- Once you understand that the forty-three muscles of the face are as affected by Parkinson's as other muscles, you have to revise the way you judge your spouse's emotional state. The best way to do so, absent smiles, winks, eyebrow motions, etc. is just to ask. And rather than saying, "You look sad/mad/miserable" or "Are you depressed?", just ask "How are you feeling?" You may often be surprised by a positive response.

- Because friends, strangers, and even doctors and other health professionals, tend to read people's moods and disposition by their faces, it is important to tell them discretely that your spouse's face may not be a good indicator of what they are feeling. Again, prompts to your spouse to tell people what they are feeling and experiencing may help people to understand that this is a book they cannot judge by its cover.

- It is possible to have speech therapy to enhance speaking, swallowing, and smiling.

Sometimes, though, particularly when taking pictures at happy times (which we all seem to do obsessively), you have to remind your spouse to "smile" and add "show your teeth."

LESSON 12: NIGHTTIME

*For most people, night is a time of rest and renewal,
however, for many people with Parkinson's disease,
night all too often brings anything but.*
—Johan Samanta, "Nighttime Parkinson's issues and
how they can be treated"

SOME YEARS AGO, my husband began to have terrifying nightmares, and reacted to them with violent physicality: screaming, sometimes falling out of the bed, and other times hitting and punching me. Once awake, he was extremely apologetic and distressed, although we both knew that none of this was intentional. Googling "sleep disturbances in Parkinson's disease" produced zero results.

The problem went on nightly for months. He would fall back to sleep immediately after the incidents, but I was usually so distraught and upset that sleep escaped me. My husband is a strong man, and Parkinson's did not make him weak; when he hit me, it hurt. I would lie there, sad and scared, wondering when it would happen again. The lack of sleep began to affect me badly. I became irritable, exhausted, depressed, and forgetful; I gained weight and hated the face that stared back at me in the mirror, pallid and weary, with ever bigger bags under my eyes.

My husband and I have slept in the same bed since we married over fifty years ago, but something had to change. He did not want me to sleep in another room, but sometimes you have to do what's best for yourself. My solution was to go to bed with him, and the first time he woke me up (which was generally two hours after we fell asleep), I moved to another, adjacent bedroom. I still heard him scream sometimes during the night, but learned to ignore it and go back to sleep.

Try as I might, at first I could find no confirmation that this issue was a symptom of Parkinson's and not unique to my husband. A report published by Suresh Kumar, et al. in 2002 concluded only that "sleep problems are much more common in PD patients compared to controls ($P < 0.001$), and correlate with increased severity of disease."[1] Thanks a lot.

A year later, a more comprehensive study by Cynthia Comella reported that "Disorders of sleep and daytime alertness are frequent in Parkinson's disease patients and arise from a number of diverse factors. The most common complaint of night-time sleep disturbance in Parkinson's disease is sleep fragmentation. Sleep fragmentation can be associated with recurrent parkinsonian symptoms, the effect of medications, concomitant medical disorders such as nocturia, or psychiatric disorders such as depression or anxiety. Likewise, nocturnal sleep disturbance may arise from sleep apnea, periodic limb movements of sleep, or rapid eye movement (REM) sleep behavior disorder."[2] Comella acknowledged also that "the presence of a sleep disturbance has consequences for both the patient and the caregiver, causing increased stress and reduced quality of life."[3]

In 2010, the Parkinson's Disease Foundation presented a one-hour online session, led by Dr. Joseph Friedman, that acknowledged that sleep problems affect 90 percent of people with Parkinson's. An article by Matthew Menza published the same year in *Movement Disorders* finally addressed the problem candidly: "Disturbances of sleep are highly prevalent in Parkinson's disease (PD), affecting up to 88 percent of community-dwelling patients. Furthermore, in studies that examine the impact on PD on quality of life (QoL), sleep difficulties are independent and important predictors of poor quality of life.... In addition, sleep disturbances contribute to excessive daytime sleepiness (EDS) and poor daytime functioning as well as patients' reduced enthusiasm for daily events. Adverse effects have also been observed in the sleep habits and the quality of life of their spousal caregivers."[4]

Finally, someone knew what we were dealing with. I no longer sleep in the same room as my husband. He doesn't like it. But it is one of the prices you have to pay for having Parkinson's. Sleep is essential for a caregiver's health, and cannot be sacrificed.

LESSON LEARNED

The sleep disturbances that accompany Parkinson's affect both the husband and the wife. Because sleep is so important to good physical and mental health, the caregiver must take whatever steps are necessary to ensure that she has a good night's slumber.

HOW TO COPE

- Be aware that sleep disturbances are very common in Parkinson's, although they may not develop until some time has passed. It is important to discuss the nature of the disordered sleep with the medical team, as there are different kinds of medication that may help.
- It is important to stick to a sleep schedule, giving evening medications as recommended by the physician, and limiting fluids.
- A Parkinson's wife is of no use to her husband if she is chronically sleep-deprived. You may need something as simple as earplugs at first, but moving to

another bedroom may be the only way you can assure yourself of a restful night. Bedrails or a baby monitor for your husband may also provide you with reassurance that he will not fall out of his bed.

LESSON 13: NO VACATIONS FOR CAREGIVERS

This is the kind of tired that sleep can't fix.

AS PARKINSON'S DISEASE PROGRESSES, you not only become a parent to your partner, but you become a single parent; not only the keeper of the house but the handyman, the decision maker, the cook, the cleaner, the nurse, the attendant. You have to mow the lawn or find someone to do it, you have to take out the trash or ask someone to help you, you have to blow the snow, wash the car, change the light bulbs, do the laundry and the dishes—in short, all the things your spouse used to do, or you used to do together. You feel like Cinderella, but it's no fairy tale.

You never get a day off. Or a week off. Or really even an hour off. There is no end in sight. I finally hired an aide for one day a week for five hours and then two days. It had gotten to the point that I could not leave him alone for even five minutes without risking a big mishap, and I had to do grocery shopping, get gas in the car, go to the dentist, meet a friend for lunch. (I know I'm being defensive, trying to justify the aides.) My primary care physician said I should hire someone five days a week for eight hours a day. But the problem is that having someone relieve you so you can run errands or even socialize doesn't eliminate the constant state of tension and worry in which you live.

The rollercoaster of emotions a Parkinson's spouse rides each and every day is grueling. They run the gamut from hope and optimism to anger and despair, but mostly seem to be negative: loneliness, helplessness, sadness. The words of Indian poet Ritu Ghatourey portray well the feelings of an exhausted Parkinson's spouse:

> "I'm tired of just not being able to live
> I'm tired of wishing for no more pain
> I'm tired of dreaming of a life I'll never have
> But most of all I'm just tired of being tired."

LESSON LEARNED

Parkinson's gives you no breaks; no weekends; no vacations. You will be tired, sometimes more tired than you ever imagined possible.

HOW TO COPE

- First and foremost, *do not feel guilty* when you get any kind of a break. Do not cut short the time you have off because you are worried about him or think that no one else can care for him they way you do. Enjoy every single minute of your freedom. You will inevitably find that he is just fine without you and maybe appreciates you more because you were away. In any case, you *deserve* the break; you work incredibly hard.

- If you can afford it, get help. If you can't afford it, maybe you can barter something you can do (Brownies? Shopping? Babysitting?) with someone who will stay with your spouse for a couple of hours. Be inventive and creative in finding ways to get out and be with others, even if you have to take him along and he is grumpy and bored when you go to a book club meeting or game of mahjong.

- Do stuff online, work on a craft project, read a great book, paint a picture, take up a hobby, plant an herb garden. There are lots of things you can do that will take your mind off your challenges and let you continue to be an interested and interesting person.

LESSON 14: THE PISA SYNDROME AND OTHER STUFF THEY DON'T TELL YOU

Empathy requires being attuned to the patient's perspective and understanding how the illness is woven into this particular person's life. Last—and this is where doctors often stumble—empathy requires being able to communicate all of this to the patient.

— Danielle Ofri, *What Doctors Feel: How Emotions Affect the Practice of Medicine*

NOT THAT I BLAME THEM. But it *would* be helpful to know. It would lessen the anxiety and the feeling that you are the only one dealing with this stuff. And it would be nice if they told you straight out, not sugarcoating it or disguising it in medical jargon, so that when it happens you are prepared and can deal with it. Even better would be coping strategies; is that asking too much?

Take the Pisa Syndrome. This is when your Parkinson's person leans over to one side. *Really* leans over, like falling-off-the-chair leaning over, or leaning on the poor person sitting next to him. Like 90-degree angle leaning over. Sure the books *mention* it (calling it "lateral trunk flexion") but they don't tell you that it can happen at any time, and that when it happens at a dinner party or a restaurant, it is not only embarrassing but makes eating impossible. And no matter how much you prop your person up, they keep leaning over. Then you find out it has a name—the Pisa Syndrome. How clever! Just like the leaning tower. Apparently it is well known: "Pisa syndrome may be a relatively frequent and often disabling complication in Parkinson's disease, especially in the advanced disease stages, according to research published in *Neurology*."[1] Really? So how come nobody mentioned it?

Like the drooling. "Excessive drooling, called sialorrhea, is a common symptom of Parkinson's and can cause awkwardness in social situations."[2] Oh yes, it definitely causes awkwardness in social situations. So again, why they don't tell you this is going to happen? Awkwardness is the least of it. People are definitely turned off by drool.

The medical people are always yakking about "off" periods and blood pressure and throw-rug hazards and grab bars. These are clear-cut issues and can be dealt with. But what about trying to have a social life with family and friends when your husband is falling off his chair and slobbering all over himself? Maybe these are not medical issues, but they are issues that have a major impact on a Parkinson's couple's social and emotional wellbeing and quality of life.

And there *are* solutions, pretty straightforward solutions. You can buy straps with Velcro that hold the patient upright. They are not the most fashion-forward accessory, but they do the job. And there are treatments for the drooling, ranging from chewing gum or hard candies to prescription eye drops under the tongue. Professional medical help is needed, but the solutions are at hand.

Why do we have to Google every symptom separately? Why don't our medical providers have booklets to give us that tell us the hard facts so that we are equipped to handle them?

LESSON LEARNED

There is a lot that you have to learn on your own. Doctors sometimes discount the non-medical problems that accompany Parkinson's.

HOW TO COPE

- This book is designed to help, as are numerous other books and online sites. The more you investigate and read, the better informed you will be.
- Sometimes you just have to ask questions. It's better to ask and find out than to

consider, wonder, and worry. You may be concerned about embarrassing your spouse if you bring up some of these issues, but just tell him in advance so he is prepared and ask. It's for his benefit, after all.

- People other than physicians may be better equipped to answer caretaking questions. Parkinson's support groups, nursing schools, health facilities may all offer talks about Parkinson's and how to deal with it, designed for the lay person. This may be a better route for getting the practical advice you need than asking the doctor.

LESSON 15: OVERWHELMED

You never know how strong you are until being strong is your only choice.
— Bob Marley

HE CAN NO LONGER DRESS himself. He can't go to the bathroom by himself. He can't cut his food. He can't sit down in a chair. He can't get up from a chair. He can feed himself sometimes, but not others. He can't sit up straight. He is at constant risk for falling. But he thinks he can do all these things; he denies any that he can't. And sometimes he can. I never know. He doesn't know what he is doing most of the time. But some of the time he does.

And of course he can always tell me how to do things, still criticize, still correct and direct. He still wants to be in charge. He is insistent on getting his way; he gets stubborn, sometimes downright nasty.

How much is him and how much is the disease? How can a man with a Ph.D. in chemistry not know how to pull down his diaper? How can he be unable to turn off a faucet, put on his slippers, turn the page in a magazine?

Why do I have to watch him every second of every minute? Every minute of every hour? The stress is unbearable. I think he actually wants me watching him; he wants me to keep him from doing dangerous things, even as he keeps doing them. He doesn't want me to yell, but how many times can I say the same thing calmly before losing it? Five, seven, nine? I can't go much beyond four. When he does the opposite of what I tell him, is he ignoring me, defying me, or is he truly unable to do what I ask? I have no idea. It is probably all of the above at one time or another.

I can't talk to him about the important things, like what we are going to do as he worsens. He is in denial about this disease. He hates having it and refuses to accommodate to it. Which means I have to make decisions by myself, and I don't feel equipped. The doctors don't help; they are not social workers. Sometimes he presents as completely normal to those who see him. I guess he makes a big effort. So is it real?

I read a novel in which a woman insisted that her husband was just faking his Parkinson's. No one was sympathetic to her position, but I understand what she was talking about. How can he be so reasonable and seemingly normal when the doctor or nurse is there, and in the next moment—when they are gone—become

drooling, blithering, helpless, demented, and hallucinating? Is it fake? Which is real? How can people who
see him in public notice in an instant how debilitated
he is, while others are taken in by his sophisticated
language and native intelligence and ignore the physical and mental symptoms? Is he one or the other or
both?

How do I know if I am dealing with Dr. Jekyll or
Mr. Hyde?

LESSON LEARNED

Parkinson's will make you confront issues you never
thought you would have to deal with, including issues
of life and death.

HOW TO COPE

- You need to have someone to talk to. A dear
  friend. A family member. A member of the
  clergy. People in a support group. A
  physician. Maybe it will be a different
  person at different times, but you need to
  have a shoulder to cry on, someone to lean
  on, a person who will listen without
  judgment and who will embrace you with
  love and understanding. Maybe you
  already know who this person is; that is
  fortunate. If you do not, it is time to start

searching, whether for professional help in the form of a therapist, or for someone in your area who is experiencing what you are. You can't do this all by yourself.

- You have to accept that your spouse is no longer the life partner he once was. His reality is now different; his thought processes are altered; his perceptions are skewed. You may still love each other deeply, but the days when you could talk about serious issues and reach consensus are over. He may make his wishes and desires clear, but decisions are ultimately up to you. Prepare yourself mentally and spiritually for this task.

- Remember also that the Parkinson's journey is not a straight one; there are bumps and detours and starts and stops along the way. He may be perfectly fine one day and psychotic the next. He may go to the doctor and get a clean bill of health and two days later be sleeping for two days straight and severely dehydrated. No one will be able to explain this for you; nobody knows. The situation is constantly changing. This is your new normal and you just have to accept it.

LESSON 16: REMARKS I COULD DO WITHOUT

Many aren't truly conscious of the words they use to "deal" with us. Some speak from a frustrated place of confusion or fear, grasping for some easy way to fix what is, at the moment, unfixable.
— Dee Kyte, *The Dumbest Things Smart People Say to Folks with MS*

"GEE, HE LOOKS GREAT!!"

You are dealing with the most awful experiences of your life. Your spouse is not the person they used to be. You are more a parent than a partner. You deal with incontinence, incoherence, paranoia. Parkinson's, particularly in the later stages, is not pretty, not easy, not pleasant. It negatively impacts every moment of your day. You are afraid to go to sleep, leave the house, even go to the bathroom, lest your spouse fall. You deal with diapers and wet beds, food spills and drool. And then some (presumably) well-meaning soul tells you your spouse "looks great!" How are you supposed to react?

I want to yell, *"It's not about looks!"* It's about where did he go? Why is his brain deteriorating? What happened to my loving, intelligent, sophisticated, talented spouse? Who can no longer read a book or a magazine, follow a conversation, watch a television program. Who can't walk without assistance, get up from a chair, follow simple directions, feed himself. And you tell me *"he looks great"*? My blood boils and my head spins and I want to holler, "You have no idea what our life is like now! We have no life! We can't go out, we can't travel, we can't go to the movies, we can't invite friends over—he is too far gone—and you tell me he 'looks great'?" But I know that that people are fishing for the only complimentary thing they can say. They can't comment on my spouse's vacant stare, lack of recognition, lack of expression, lack of interest, lack of language. So they say, "He looks great!" and I hear myself reply, "Thank you."

The second hurtful thing people say without thinking is "I hope he is better." *No*, he is *not better*. He will never be better. He will only get worse. Parkinson's is a downhill slide and there are no stop signs along the route. I'm a relatively cheerful person, and I try to be as upbeat and positive as I can about this journey, but it is not a voyage of discovery or a happy camping trip. I have no problem with people who ask how my husband is doing and I won't dump my anguish upon them. I'll say "okay" or "as well as can be expected" and move on.

But to ask if he is *better* is to totally misunderstand the situation and to imply that if he is not better, then someone isn't doing a good job. Parkinson's is an illness, sure, but it's not the flu or the common cold. It doesn't improve. A better thing to say is, "I hope your husband is well" and let it go at that. At least you're not stabbing the spouse in the heart.

LESSON LEARNED

Most people know little to nothing about Parkinson's; this includes some health care professionals.

HOW TO COPE

- You have to educate people. You don't have to lose your cool or get angry, but you have to explain that Parkinson's means more than a hand tremor, that it affects every aspect of the patient's life, including his ability to speak, react, smile, eat, walk, etc. People are uncomfortable around those with Parkinson's, in part because there is less responsiveness than with other people. You may have to subtly remind them that your husband is still there, and if they give him a chance and time, he will show them.

- Because people with Parkinson's tend to react and respond slowly, because their faces do not reveal their emotions or their comprehension of a conversation, many health professionals will direct their attention to you, the spouse, who seems more actively engaged with them. Do not allow them to do this. Make them speak directly to your husband and ask questions to be sure he understands. It may take a little longer, but it's important for them to respect your husband's dignity and his role in his medical treatments.

- Accept that you can't change everything and everyone. "Forgive them, for they know not what they do" is a good adage for dealing with people who say things that are irksome to you. They mean well, after all.

LESSON 17: I WANT TO SCREAM

Sometimes I feel like throwing in the towel.
But you know what that means... More laundry.

PEOPLE CAN BE SO CRUEL. My husband and I were returning from Florida, where we escape two months of the wintry Syracuse weather. (It's *really* hard to push a wheelchair in knee-deep snow.) The woman at airport security scrutinized our driver's licenses. She looked at my husband and then at the photo on his ID. "You should get a new picture of him," she remarked sourly. "And you should get Parkinson's," I screamed .... but silently, to myself, because I was too well-bred to scream it at her. But I wanted to, oh, how I wanted to.

I want to scream a lot. I want to scream when I am pushing a wheelchair into a movie theater and the person in front of me doesn't hold the door open. I want to scream when I go to a restaurant and there's no way to enter that doesn't involve stairs or double doors. I want to scream when I dress my husband and half an hour later, he takes his clothes off. Or when I change his diaper and fifteen minutes later, he has a bowel movement. I want to scream when he wakes me up four nights in a row at 5:00 A.M. And I want to scream when he decides to try to take a shower when I dash out to the ATM.

There are a lot of times I want to scream. And there are a lot of times I *do* scream. I'm not proud of it; I'm ashamed of it. I know it's not his fault that he wakes me up in the middle of the night to change his diaper or that I have to repeat *the exact same things* over and over every day, several times a day (*"Lift your foot, point your toe down; now the other foot, point your toe down; now pull the pants up." "Hold the arm of the chair, turn around and sit down slowly." "Stand up straight, take big steps, heel first."*) But frustration, exhaustion, sleep deprivation, and the endlessness of it all take a toll on one's patience. Especially if one is not a particularly patient person to begin with.

So I scream. Mostly silently. Mostly to my pillow. Sometimes, to my shame, at my husband. Strangely, though he doesn't like it, he quickly forgets it. And I'm getting better. Screaming is useless, except as a way of letting off steam. It doesn't make anything better. I don't want to be told that it's wrong to scream, and I don't want to be absolved of guilt for screaming. I just need to learn how to cope without losing it. Maybe I'll buy a screaming pillow on Amazon.

LESSON LEARNED

Nobody's perfect.

HOW TO COPE

- Some people are born caregivers. They delight in taking care of others and the very act of caretaking makes them happy. Other people are different. They do not find the tasks associated with caregiving to be fulfilling. Unfortunately, Parkinson's does not afflict only people whose spouses relish the care partner role. If you fall into the second category, recognize it, own it—and then do your level best to care for your spouse as well as you can. You don't have a choice, so make the best of it. In time, as you gain experience and become better at it, you may find that it has its rewards.
- Find a way to blow off steam. There are times when you will become exasperated and angry. This is normal. Do whatever it takes to vent your emotions in a safe way—and don't direct your anger at your spouse. Yell your head off in the basement, run on your treadmill, knead some dough, hammer some nails, scrub out the refrigerator. Or do

some yoga or a meditation exercise.
Whatever works for you.

- Spend ten minutes a day in nature. Being
outdoors for even a short time reduces
stress and anger. Nature is a restorative
environment, which has been proven to be
calming and therapeutic. It is an antidote to
anger and an effective therapy, even in
small doses. Watching the clouds, listening
to the birds, feeling the breeze, enjoying a
sunset, smelling the morning air, even
shivering in the cold helps us relax and put
our problems in better perspective.

LESSON 18: THE IMAGINARY
BOYFRIEND

James Parkinson, in his famous 1817 Essay on the
Shaking Palsy, *portrayed the disease that now bears his
name as one that affected movement and posture, while
leaving the senses and the intellect unimpaired. And in
the century-and-a-half that followed, there was virtually
no mention of perceptual disorders or hallucinations in
patients with Parkinson's disease.*
— Oliver Sacks, *Hallucinations*

HIS NAME apparently is Tim and he is a musician in a
band. He drives a white sports car. He comes to visit
each night between 2:00 and 4:00 A.M. My husband
knows this because he hears him, but when he goes to
investigate, Tim disappears into holes in the floor
leading to tunnels that go outside. My husband says I
married Tim in a ceremony in the basement, attended
by fifty to one hundred people. Tim smokes. He does

not have a job. Some of the friends who attended the wedding followed us to Florida, where my husband saw a couple of them in a parking lot (they disappeared when he pointed them out to me). My husband hates Tim with a passion and asks me what I see in him. I cannot answer *because Tim does not exist.*

This might appear harmless except that it is not. One day my husband and I were sitting not two feet from each other on the balcony of the Florida apartment we rent. Suddenly, my husband stood up and went inside. I could see he was very upset. "What's the matter?" I asked. "You call yourselves Christians!" he exploded. "You're pagans! I won't stand for this!" Completely taken aback, I asked what he was talking about. He then accused me of performing a sexual act with Tim on the balcony. No matter what I said, no matter what arguments I advanced about the absurdity of the charge, he refused to let go of it. He was furious for two days. "I know what I saw," he insisted. It's very scary.

Turns out there is another syndrome associated with Parkinson's. It's called the Othello Syndrome. It is defined as "a type of paranoid delusional jealousy, characterized by the false absolute certainty of the infidelity of a partner, leading to preoccupation with a partner's sexual unfaithfulness based on unfounded evidence."[1] Do you know how terrifying it is when your husband screams at you with unbridled hatred and accusations of the vilest type? Do you know how reassuring it is when you learn that there is something called the

Othello Syndrome and that it is caused by the disease and not by anything you did or anything he thought he saw or heard?

I have not found the Othello Syndrome mentioned in any of the many books I have read about Parkinson's. I happened upon some academic studies while Googling things like "accusations of infidelity in Parkinson's" or some such topic. I had seen references to paranoia and accusations of infidelity, but never anything as clear and definitive as this. I believe that knowledge is power, and the power of this knowledge has totally altered the way I react to his continuing belief in the existence of Tim and my supposed relationship to him. I will print out the article to show him, but it really doesn't matter if it doesn't convince him that he is wrong. I now recognize that the accusations are part of the disease process and I'm better able to handle them with something approaching equanimity.

LESSON LEARNED

Dementia is the worst part of Parkinson's. Fifty to eighty percent of people with Parkinson's will develop dementia, and ten years is the average time from diagnosis until the onset of dementia. Nobody wants to tell you this.

HOW TO COPE

- Be prepared. Dementia is something that is more likely than not to affect your spouse. When you begin to see signs of thought impairment, you will have to change how you interact and you will have to be alert to keep both you and your husband safe. Where once you thought nothing of leaving him alone in the house while you ran an errand, that may no longer be advisable. Where before he paid the bills, you may now find that you are getting notices threatening to cut off your electricity or your car insurance. Little by little, and without making a fuss, you will have to take over aspects of your life that were previously his domain. Preparation is the key to making this transition successful.
- If hallucinations and delusions become severe, tell his physician. There are effective medications for these problems, but they have to be administered carefully with close observation of the results. You don't want your husband to be a zombie; you just want him to stop seeing people and animals that aren't there.
- Stay calm. Things that are nonexistent for you are very real to him. And often very

scary. You need to calmly reassure him that his mind is playing tricks on him. Allow him to approach or try to touch the hallucinations to prove that they aren't there. If he believes you are unfaithful, reassure him that you love him. But most importantly, try not to overreact. You know none of this is real, but he doesn't. You just have to accept that fact.

LESSON 19: VARIABILITY

Parkinson's is a slow but inevitable process. It's hard living with it on a daily basis. The difficulty facing people with it is that they never quite know "Can I or can't I do this today?"
— Helen Mirren, "It's Time We All Understood Parkinson's Disease"

THEY SAY that the two big unknowns for people with Parkinson's are the rate of disease progression and the extent of affliction. But another one of the astonishing things about Parkinson's is its variability, not only from person to person but within one person. When I read blogs by people with Parkinson's, I am amazed at the variety of ways the disease manifests itself. There are those who have lost the ability to speak (though they still write well) and others who are running marathons after deep brain stimulation surgery. There are those who go to the gym regularly and others who are wheelchair-bound, those who continue to work and those who go on disability. This is not a matter of choice. Some people can do things and others cannot, and all the medication and physical therapy in the world cannot halt the inexorable progress of the illness.

But even more astounding to me is the capriciousness and unpredictability of the manifestations of Parkinson's within a single individual, within a single day, within an hour, within minutes. In my husband's case, on some days he can get up, stand straight, and walk normally, without the walker. On others, he cannot get out of bed without assistance, and ambulation consists of tiny little stutter-steps as he holds onto the walker for dear life with a posture that resembles a bent pretzel. There is no causation or consistency involved—no change in medication, activity, sleep, eating, stress. Sometimes he can and sometimes he can't.

Some days we are having a conversation and he will suddenly ask me about the other person in the room, lowering his voice to a whisper. There is no other person in the room. Or when he is sitting next to me at the table and suddenly asks, "Where is Barbara?" When I ask, "What did you say?" he says, "Oh! There you are." Or when he jumps up from his chair and heads for the stairs, announcing, "I have to go to the framer" to put glass in two picture frames that are thirty years old. Ten minutes later, this is all in the past and forgotten.

I have learned (slowly) not to react, but it is a challenge. How is it that some days he can comment articulately on world events, and a few minutes later be seeing cats and dogs that aren't there? How is it that he can read scientific magazines and discuss their contents one minute and an hour later not be able to read a menu? Some days he can eat his lunch and other days he needs to be fed because he cannot get a mouthful on the fork?

I guess the answer is the one given to me by a wise physician friend: sometimes the synapses work, and sometimes they don't. One has to adjust, but it is bizarre and unsettling.

LESSON LEARNED

The one thing you can predict about Parkinson's is that it will be unpredictable.

HOW TO COPE

- Before you react to anything, count slowly to ten. Consider your response. Remember that you are dealing with a person with a neurodegenerative disease, not just a normal person. Remind yourself that he cannot help what he is doing or not doing. It is the disease, not him, that is causing him to shake, fall, speak so softly you cannot hear him, hallucinate, be incontinent, unable to eat or read or write his name. It's not a nice disease, so even though he could do it yesterday, it doesn't mean he can do it today. Counting to ten will give you time to remember this.

- Just as you should not compare his today with his yesterday or make assumptions about tomorrow, neither should you compare him to any other person with Parkinson's. People frequently tell you of others, who had deep brain stimulation or who work out every day or who work or who are in a nursing home—whatever they tell you is meaningless, because it's apples and oranges. Parkinson's affects people differently and it moves in stages. Even people at the same stage are affected differently. There are no generalizations or comparisons to be made. Every individual is unique. You may have to remind others of this fact.

- Live in the moment. If it is a good day, and he can move well and is feeling well, then enjoy it to the hilt. Do something fun together and appreciate it for what it is. Don't make plans to do it again the next day or the next week. He may crash from exhaustion or may simply be unable to move. Just live each day to the fullest. There will be good days and bad days, so take full advantage of those good days whenever they happen.

LESSON 20: YOU HAVE TO LAUGH

Always laugh when you can. It is cheap medicine.
— Lord Byron

THEY SAY that every time you find some humor in a difficult situation, you win. Take these actual discussions with my husband.

"Hon, would you please put out water for the dog and the cat?" he asked.

"We don't have a dog or a cat," I said.

"But the cat is right over there."

"No, it isn't. You're having a hallucination."

"Oh. Okay. But what about the water?"

"I'm not putting out water for an imaginary dog and cat.... Oh, never mind. I'll put out imaginary water."

Or, at a different time: "Why do you have a cat on your head?" he asked.

"I don't have a cat on my head."

"Oh."

Later that day, a man climbs a tree in our backyard to trim it.

"What is that guy doing?" he asked.

"He's looking for the cat."

"Oh."

Some people might think it cruel to laugh at situations like these, but if you can't laugh, you can't survive. Even my husband can see the humor.

The hallucinations aren't always funny. When he sees a bride in the backyard, or a cow on the lawn, or an elephant in the road, it's pretty clear that it's a Parkinson's symptom. But when he believes that his very faithful wife (me) has a lover who sneaks in the house at 2:00 A.M. and then leaves in his white sports car every night, it hurts. And when, in his search for the lover, he shines a flashlight in my face while I'm asleep, it's irritating. And when he goes racing around the house day and night looking for the holes in the floor which allow the lover to escape, it goes beyond hurtful and irritating to dangerous, because of the risk of falls.

A great deal of protestation on my part does something to alleviate his delusion, but he still is not totally convinced. When I read him the passage from Dr. Friedman's book that says that Parkinson's frequently causes sufferers to believe that their spouse is unfaithful, he is somewhat relieved. And when we talk to the neurologist, who recommends a medication adjustment, the symptoms temporarily subside, even without upping the dosage.

You have to laugh, otherwise you will cry.

I arrange for my daughter to stay with my husband and tell him where I am going.

"I'm going to the funeral for Anne's husband," I say.

"Oh. What's the matter with him?"

"He's dead."

LESSON LEARNED

Parkinson's isn't funny, but life can still be funny if you have Parkinson's.

HOW TO COPE

- Make comedy and humor a big part of your life. No matter how disabled a person becomes, being able to laugh is always uplifting. In fact, laughter really is good medicine (it releases dopamine) and laughing at television programs, comedy shows, or movies will provide both you and your spouse with a shared and enjoyable experience. You'll be amazed at how much pleasure you will get out of seeing your spouse laugh.
- Don't be afraid to laugh at the ways

Parkinson's has affected your life. It doesn't all have to be doom and gloom. There *are* aspects of life with Parkinson's that are funny, and it's important to recognize them. Invite people over to help you keep things in perspective; young children especially help you to see things in a unique way. Example: Our youngest granddaughter, three years old, called my husband's lift chair "The Rocket Ship." He retorted, "It's the Electric Chair."

- They say that learning to laugh at yourself is fundamental to good mental health. When you get distraught at the myriad challenges of caregiving, step back and find the humor in your situation. Maybe it's as simple as reading the consoling words on a sign for the laundry room that reads:

SOMETIMES YOU MIGHT FEEL LIKE NO ONE'S THERE FOR YOU, BUT YOU KNOW WHO'S ALWAYS THERE FOR YOU?

LAUNDRY. LAUNDRY WILL ALWAYS BE THERE FOR YOU.

I'm sleep deprived. I'm overwhelmed. I'm overweight, because I eat my stress. I can't keep up with anything. I have depression, high cholesterol and blood pressure, and sleep apnea. I see a therapist and psychiatrist.
— Amy Ridout, PillPack.com, "What Happens To A Marriage After Parkinson's"

THESE WORDS BY JAN, a Parkinson's wife, ring so true to me. Food is now my best friend. It comforts me and fills me and sustains me. It keeps me overweight, but it doesn't judge and it doesn't pity and it doesn't avoid me. Not that my friends aren't wonderful, but I know that if I share my life, my problems, my angst, my fears with them, they will be discomfited and, unable to help, will turn away to pleasanter things and other more cheerful companions.

Caregivers can place unrealistic demands on themselves. They want their involvement to have a positive effect on the health and happiness of the person with Parkinson's. Unfortunately, this is magical thinking. Parkinson's is a progressive neurodegenerative disease, and the most talented and compassionate caregiver cannot impact its trajectory.

So I wake up each morning with a sense of dread. If he woke me during the night, at least I know he's alive. I know Parkinson's won't kill him in his sleep, but I can't help worrying that it will. So I wake up and I listen. Do I hear/see breathing? Snoring? Anything? Then comes the waiting. When will he wake up? Some days it's 6:00 A.M., others it's noon. There's no consistency. Will he be able to get out of bed by himself or call for help? Will he be hungry or not? Eat breakfast or not? Go back to bed or not? So you sit around and wait to see what the morning has in store for you. You can't make plans because your life is too unpredictable. You are always, always, always on call.

The dementia makes things worse. A British study found that, for caregivers, "cognitive impairment has a greater emotional impact than the physical symptoms associated with [Parkinson's disease]. Central to emotional distress in carers were feelings of loss of their loved one, helplessness, and feeling overwhelmed by cognitive impairment and associated symptoms."[1] The researchers found that hallucinations, delusions, and outbursts of aggression were not recognized by the person with Parkinson's but were "evidently distressing for the carers and challenging to cope with" because they were disruptive, unpredictable, and distressing. I certainly found this to be the case. When my husband was accusing me of infidelity, when he thought he was President of the United States and people were coming to shoot him, it did me little good to know that half of people with Parkinson's also develop Parkinson's disease psychosis. As upset as I was by the absurd accusations of infidelity and the understanding that he was delusional about the presidency, what I was most distressed about was—how do you communicate with a person who is so far removed from reality?

Hope is a powerfully sustaining force for people who are ill and for their caregivers, but it can also be detrimental. Each time I see a flash of my husband's intelligence or awareness, I unconsciously assume that things are better. But they're not. I know this, but I still delude myself. I am not alone in this. Caregivers frequently overestimate the intellectual ability of their patients. Caregivers are people-pleasers; they are compassionate; they *care*. But sometimes they can be their own worst enemies. Our need to make people happy and to make things better may actually do the opposite. Take falling, for instance. Falls are among the leading causes of death in people with Parkinson's. In my concern over the possibility (read: likelihood) of my husband falling, I continually remind him to slow down, use the walker, take big steps, don't walk on tiptoe, straighten up. In short, I nag. Nag, nag, nag. Does it help? Of course not. As Dr. Friedman writes, "Nagging is demoralizing for the nagger and the one being nagged. The nagger feels ignored and the one being nagged feels misunderstood or morally weak, as if not trying hard enough."[2]

A Parkinson's husband hit the nail on the head when he wrote, "If you choose to be the primary caregiver for your spouse, you will find it is one of the most demanding tasks you've ever tackled. It is a major commitment, and not one to be taken lightly." I think the hardest part, and the reason I wrote this book, is the aloneness. Although I have never wanted to join a support group, I find tremendous consolation when I discover that my experiences are not just mine alone. Take yelling, for instance. My husband often tells me to "stop yelling." Inevitably, I reply, "I'm not yelling." And I don't think I am. I think I am just enunciating or speaking up so he will hear me. But to him, it's yelling. And maybe it is. Maybe what he is picking up on is not the volume of my voice, but my tone. And maybe that tone reflects emotions that I am not hiding well. That is why it was so helpful to me to read the words of another Parkinson's wife, Jan Rabinowitz, who wrote, "Patience is very difficult to come by when interacting with Allen. He is often telling me to stop yelling at him. But yelling is what I do first [when I'm scared]: when he falls, for instance."[3]

Another research finding that rings true to me is the need caregivers have for appreciation. "Spending time attempting to provide help can be beneficial for a caregiver's mental and physical well-being,' wrote Dr. Michael Poulin, professor of psychology at the University at Buffalo, "but only during those times when the caregiver sees that their help has made a difference and that difference is noticed and recognized by their partner."[4] As I operate at the limit of my patience and stamina, only to be met with surliness or resistance, I often feel my resentment and anger building up. "If only he'd appreciate what I'm doing for him," I think, "it would make this whole business so much easier." It's not that I expect thanks for every little thing, or candy and flowers. But it would be nice if, just once in a while, he recognized and acknowledged what I do with an expression of appreciation. And sometimes, at odd moments, he does.

But sometimes I just need a kick in the pants. In a book chock full of suggestions on how to make caregiving for Parkinson's go more smoothly, Lianna Marie wrote one sentence that completely resonated with me. If you're struggling with mixed feelings about your spouse and your marriage, it's okay, she said: "Don't beat yourself up about it."[5] This is great advice. Get over it. Sometimes when I'm wallowing in self-pity, I need to be reminded that this is not the worst thing that could happen to anybody, that other people have it a lot worse. I'm not the one with Parkinson's. Caregiving is what I do, but it's not what I am. There are still lots of reasons for me—and my husband—to be happy to get up every morning, even if I'm exhausted by the time night falls.

In writing this book, my hope is that it will give other Parkinson's spouses some valuable signposts on their own Parkinson's journeys, from someone who's been there. I hope I have provided some things to reflect on, some coping strategies to make this life somewhat easier, and perhaps a chuckle or two. The Parkinson's wife has a tough road, but as Eleanor Roosevelt pointed out, "A woman is like a tea bag—you can't tell how strong she is until you put her in hot water."

Research has found that, for some, being a Parkinson's spouse has made them "more patient, understating, and resilient as a result of caring for a loved one."[6] Most of us rise to meet the challenges of being a Parkinson's partner and survive, learning as we go along, and growing from strength to strength. As someone once said, a strong woman knows she has strength enough for the journey, but a woman of strength knows it is in the journey where she will become strong.

ABOUT THE AUTHOR

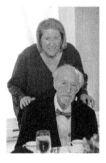 Barbara Sheklin Davis, a graduate of Barnard College, has an M.A. and Ph.D. from Columbia University. She is Professor Emerita of Modern Languages at Onondaga Community College and served as principal of the Syracuse Hebrew Day School for twenty-seven years. She has written two books of local history: *Syracuse African Americans* and *The Syracuse Jewish Community* (with Susan Rabin). More recently, she examined aspects of the Jewish world in three books: *100 Jewish Things to Do Before You Die*; *A Parallel Universe: Haredi Women Leading Haredi Schools for Girls* (with Zipora Schorr); and *Two Jews Three Opinions: Klal Yisrael, Pluralism and the Jewish Community Day School Network*. She and her husband, Dr. Leslie Davis, are the proud parents of three children and grandparents of nine.

END NOTES

LESSON 3: CLINGING

1. Sheri Samotin, "Strategies for Dealing with a 'Clingy' Senior," https://www.agingcare.com/articles/how-to-handle-a-clingy-senior-163600.htm

LESSON 4: DOCTOR VISITS

1. https://www.kevinmd.com/blog/2015/11/what-worries-me-about-husbands-and-wives-in-the-exam-room.html

LESSON 6: GUILT

1. Lisa Hutchison, "Releasing Resentment" https://caregiver.com/articles/releasing-resentment .
2. Elizz, "Kicking Family Caregiver Guilt To The Curb," https://elizz.com/caregiver-resources/just-for-caregivers/dealing-with-caregiver-guilt

LESSON 11: IS THERE SOMEBODY IN THERE?

1. Sherri Woodbridge, "Don't Judge Me by the Absence of My Smile," https://parkinsonsnewstoday.com/2018/05/23/people-parkinsons-shouldnt-judged-smile/
2. Matt Townsend, "Communicating With The People Who Don't Emote," https://www.matttownsend.com/2016/05/09/communicating-with-the-people-who-dont-emote/

LESSON 12: NIGHTTIME

1. Suresh Kuman, et al, "Sleep disorders in Parkinson's disease," https://www.ncbi.nlm.nih.gov/pubmed/12210875

2. Cynthia Comella, "Sleep disturbances in Parkinson's disease," https://www.ncbi.nlm.nih.gov/pubmed/12583848

3. Ibid.

4. Matthew Menza, et al. "Sleep Disturbances in Parkinson's Disease," https://onlinelibrary.wiley.com/doi/abs/10.1002/mds.22788

LESSON 14: THE PISA SYNDROME AND OTHER STUFF THEY DON'T TELL YOU

1. MDEdge.com, https://www.mdedge.com/neurology/article/105366/movement-disorders/pisa-syndrome-may-be-relatively-common-complication

2. Parkinson's Foundation, https://www.parkinson.org/Understanding-Parkinsons/Symptoms/Movement-Symptoms/Drooling

LESSON 18: THE IMAGINARY BOYFRIEND

1. Hiroshi Kataoka and Kazuma Sugie, *Delusional Jealousy (Othello Syndrome) in 67 Patients with Parkinson's Disease, https://www.ncbi.nlm.nih.gov/pmc/articles/PMC5845894/*

EPILOGUE

1. Rachael A. Lawson, Daniel Collerton, John-Paul Taylor, David J. Burn, and Katie R. Brittain, *Coping with Cognitive Impairment in People with Parkinson's Disease and Their Carers: A Qualitative Study,* https://www.hindawi.com/journals/pd/2018/1362053/

2. Friedman, p. 208

3. https://folks.pillpack.com/what-happens-to-a-marriage-after-parkinsons/

4. Michael J. Poulin, Joan K. Monin, Stephanie L. Brown, Kenneth M. Langa. "Spouses' Daily Feelings of Appreciation and Self-Reported Well-Being," *Health Psychology*, 2017; DOI: 10.1037/hea0000527

5. Lianne Marie, *Everything You Need to Know About Caregiving for Parkinson's Disease*, p. 123

6. N. R. Netto, G. Y. N. Jenny, and Y. L. K. Philip, "Growing and gaining through caring for a loved one with dementia," *Dementia*, vol. 8, no. 2, pp. 245–261, 2009